Foreword

I can't help but wonder at how amazing the human body is. It really is the crowning achievement of the universe. At its heart is your cosmic interface, the nervous system. The nervous system helps us interact with the beautiful world around us and maintain health and balance within ourselves. It is truly a treasure that we must honor and use to live our best lives. Our brain connects and regulates our body functions through the spinal cord, peripheral nerves, and an information highway called the vagus nerve.

It is no easy task to regulate the function of over 60 trillion cells around the clock, but somehow it is happening right now. Millions of signals are spreading to and from the brain, reaching all organs and systems in your body and keeping your systems and life in balance. They let you breathe, digest, regenerate, repair, reproduce, and regulate. All this is thanks to the vagus nerve.

As we continue to unlock the secrets of the horizon above us and the vastness within us, it is difficult not to live in a constant state of awe and wonder at human potential. That's why I'm so happy that you're devoting yourself to this book. I am sure that this book will bring you closer to unleashing your best possible life!

As you will learn, this knowledge has been applied in all forms of Eastern medicine for thousands of years. You may wonder why no one has ever told you about the simple solutions described in this book. The reason may shock you at first, but it will become quite clear as you begin to pay attention to the clues around you. The allopathic model of health care works under a model that believes your body is making mistakes and does not know how to regulate itself and that there is nothing you can do.

Using this framework and convincing others (through marketing) that this is the case, millions of people have been made to take prescription drugs, mutilate their wonderful bodies, and poison their minds.

Vagus Nerve for Beginners

How to improve your heart rate, liver function, blood sugar, and much more through vagus nerve exercises and meditation techniques

Marvin Kunz

1st edition

2019

Table of contents

As a result, medical costs have skyrocketed, drug dependency has increased, and no results have been achieved. The patient's body is not seen as a partner in the healing journey, but as the cause of disease. Nothing could be further from the truth.

In the vitalist model of health, we work under a completely different paradigm. We believe that all your body parts are needed, that your body can regulate itself and that you can only be healthy if you follow the laws of nature. We believe that, as a human being, you have an innate healing potential that is stronger than any measure known to man. We believe that nothing can heal your body better than itself.

But here is the key: Only you can do the work described on these pages. Only you!

You have been blessed with this amazing life, and this book will help you to live it.

The science behind it all: what is the vagus nerve?

Anatomists were perplexed. How can a single nerve that starts in the brain stem be so long and connect to so many different organs? What effects could this nerve have? With so many possible functions, what would happen if this nerve were injured or severed?

How's the vagus nerve?

The vagus nerve (VN) has its origin in the brain, essentially the brain stem, which records, processes and regulates the vast majority of the body's automatic functions. Most of the time we do not have to consciously think about these functions to realize them. These functions are called autonomic functions and are regulated by your autonomic nervous system.

Why is it called the vagus nerve?

Vagus is derived from a Latin word that means "to wander, to roam, to walk" and to a lesser extent "uncertain or vague". Because of the large and unspecific nature of the nerve, the anatomists and researchers wanted a descriptive word that meant exactly that. When they came upon the word vagus, they essentially called this nerve "the wanderer".

Some of the functions that are regulated by the autonomic nervous system are

- Heartbeat
- blinking of the eyelids
- Respiratory rate and deep
- vasoconstriction and dilation
- Detoxification in liver and kidneys
- Digestion in the digestive tract
- Opening and closing of the sweat glands
- Saliva production and tearing
- pupil dilation and constriction

- Urination

Inside the brain stem are various clusters of neuron cell bodies called nuclei. This is where neurons take up information from other cells throughout the body. These nuclei have different functions and are distinguished by Latin names. Nuclei are like a router with a home Internet network connection.

Some information comes into the router through the cable connection or telephone line, the information is processed in the router, and other information is then sent from the router to your computer, TV, and any other electronics connected to your network. There are two main types of neurons and they send information in one of two directions. The first is afferent neurons, which receive information about what is happening in and around the body. Afferent neurons take information from the body towards the brain, which is called afferent information.

The second are called efferent neurons, which send information with regulatory or motor effects (so-called efferent information) to various organs and structures throughout the body so that efferent information is transmitted from the brain to the body. The vagus nerve is connected to four different nuclei in the brain stem. Eighty percent of the information transmitted by the UN is afferent information, which means that the most common direction in which information flows in the UN is from the organs of the body to the brain.

The remaining 20 percent of neurons in the UN have an efferent signal from the brain to the body that leads to specific functions in each cell and organ. It is fascinating to know that most medical students are shocked to learn that only 20 percent of UN function is efferent because it has so many efferent effects on the organs. Just imagine how much information this nerve returns to the brain, more than four times as much as the information it transmits from it.

Like the wires of your home network connection, the bundles of neurons in your nerves send information about their length using electrical signals that, once they reach the nerve endings, result in the release of a chemical signal called a neurotransmitter. These neurotransmitters bind to receptors on the recipient cells, which results in an effect in the cells at the end of the connection. The main neurotransmitter used by the UN is called acetylcholine, which has a strong anti-inflammatory effect in the body.

The management of the inflammatory system is one of the most important functions of the UN. It is the most important inflammatory control system in the body and has far-reaching effects on your health and diseases. Many of the health conditions that patients suffer from are due to high rates of inflammation in certain organs and systems, from the digestive tract to the liver and brain.

Inflammation is an important reaction in the body to protect us from bacterial and viral invaders, physical trauma and other things that ideally should not enter the body. If the inflammation levels are not kept in check and progress chronically, the effects can be many and varied, leading to many different health problems. Some common conditions that correlate with high levels of inflammation include

- Alzheimer
- Arthritis
- Asthma
- Cancer
- Crohn's disease
- Diabetes
- cardiovascular diseases
- High blood pressure
- High cholesterol level
- Orthostatic tachycardia syndrome (POTS)
- colitis ulcerosa

Most of the organs affected by these diseases are stimulated (or linked) by the UN. So it is not only possible but very likely that the UN will not work suboptimally and will not have its anti-inflammatory effect on these organs, leading to chronic inflammation and disease. It is important to remember that these conditions do not occur in isolation and if one of these conditions is present, it is likely that another will occur.

The same signals are sent through the vagus nerve to and from almost every internal organ, so the same thing will likely happen in other areas if the rate of inflammation in one organ is not controlled.

Where is the vagus nerve located?

The vagus nerve is the longest nerve in the body. Without getting too technical, I would like to explain where the nerve begins and how it reaches the organs it innervates and provides with information. Let us follow its course through the body.

Brain stem connections

The neurons that form the vagus nerve begin in the brainstem and come from four different nuclei. These nuclei consist of the dorsal vagus nucleus, the solitaire nucleus, the trigeminal spinal nerve, and the ambiguous nucleus. Each of these nuclei controls specific component fibers of the nerve.

Sensory neurons deliver signals from the skin, which the vagus nerve transmits to the spinal trigeminal nucleus. This includes a certain part of the skin of the ear, which is important for the activation of the vagus nerve by acupuncture. Signals from the internal organs of the body are brought to the solitary core via the vagus nerve and are transported to the brain for further processing. These signals include signals from the stomach, digestive tract, lungs, heart, liver, gall bladder, pancreas, and spleen.

We are also able to send direct signals to these organs through the vagus nerve by using parasympathetic fibers originating in the dorsal vagus nucleus. These signals help to calm and regulate the function of the heart and lungs and increase the effect of the intestines and digestive tract, liver, pancreas, gall bladder, and spleen. The final nucleus that contributes fibers to the UN is the nucleus ambiguus. This nucleus sends out neurons that have a motor function specifically aimed at controlling the majority of muscles in the neck and upper airways.

These muscles are responsible for keeping the airways open and using the vocal cords to produce sound and thus create your voice. The right and left vagus are the only nerves in the body with four different functions and four different nuclei that specifically contribute component fibers. Most other nerves in the body carry simple sensory information from the skin and motor signals for movement to the muscles. This simple distinction should show you how important the vagus nerve is and how extensive its function is. Let us now follow the path of the nerves from the brain stem down to the neck, thorax (chest area) and abdomen (abdominal area).

In the throat

From the area of the brain stem known as the medulla oblongata, the fibers of the left and right vagus nerves extend into the cranial cavity (the inside of the skull) and converge to form what we call the vagus nerve. The nerve then exits the skull through an opening called the jugular foramen. This opening is a large space for the nerve and other blood vessels that run between the neck and skull.

As soon as the VN exits the skull, it enters the upper cervical area just behind the ear, between the internal jugular vein and the internal carotid artery. These blood vessels are the direct bloodlines to and from the brain and are extremely important in keeping us alive. The proximity to these specific blood vessels is an indication of how important the vagus nerve is, as physical damage to any of these three structures can cause irreparable damage.

Damage to blood vessels can lead directly to death, while damage to the nerve leads to complete dysfunction in many organs of the body. Immediately after the vagus has passed the jugular foramen, the nerve thickens, which is called the superius ganglion (or jugular ganglion).

A ganglion is a thickening of a nerve formed by an accumulation of sensory neuron cell bodies that are in very close proximity to each other. The cell bodies of the sensory nerves gather in this ganglion and then re-form into the thinner nerve section from which the first branch of the vagus nerve emerges.

The first branch of the UN is called the auricular branch. The auricular branch goes through an opening, the mastoid canal, back into the skull and to the ear through another hole in the skull, the tympanomastoid cleft. The nerve extends to the skin of each ear. This branch senses touch, temperature, and moisture on the skin of the ear, especially the outer canal, tragus, and pinna. It is the main target for activating the treatment for VN dysfunction with auricular acupuncture (acupuncture points in the ear).

When the nerve begins to migrate down from the superius ganglion (or inferius, in anatomical language), the UN becomes thicker again and forms the inferior ganglion. This ganglion contains the cell bodies of the neurons that are involved in receiving information from the internal organs. The nerve then thins out again and immediately enters a passage that is created by a thickening of the connective tissue, the so-called carotid artery.

Together with the internal carotid artery and the internal jugular vein, the vagus nerve receives additional soft tissue protection when it passes through the neck. In the carotid artery, the vagus nerve releases its next branch: the pharyngeal branch. The pharyngeal branch contains neurons from the vagus nerve, but also some contributing neurons from the ninth and eleventh cranial nerves (lingual nerve and accessorius nerve). As these neurons converge, they move towards the midline of the body until they reach the upper part of the neck, called the pharynx. In the throat, the vagus nerve transmits movement signals to several muscles involved in the swallowing reflex, controlling the opening and closing of the upper airways and maintaining the gag reflex.

When the vagus nerve descends the sides of the neck within the carotid artery, the third branch, called the recurrent nerve, is formed. This nerve branches from the VN shortly after the pharyngeal branch and delivers motor signals to the muscles of the larynx above the vocal cords, especially to the muscles that control the pitch of your voice. As the VN moves down through the carotid artery, it creates the cervical branches of the heart, which are two of the three branches that penetrate the heart.

The third branch, the thoracic branch of the heart, develops shortly after leaving the carotid artery in the chest area (thorax). These branches mix with the nerves of the sympathetic nervous system and form the cardiac plexus (a plexus, pluralized as a plexi, is a collection of mixing nerve fibers of different branches and nerves of different origins that develop to a specific location). We have two cardiac plexuses: one in front of the aorta, called the plexus cardiacus superficalis, and one behind the arch of the aorta, called the plexus cardiacus profundus.

(The aorta is the primary blood vessel that carries blood from the heart to the rest of the body). Some fibers of the cardiac plexus extend towards the sinoatrial (SA) node of the heart, while others extend towards the atrioventricular (AV) node. We will discuss the function of these nerves at the heart in the next chapter. For now, it is most important to remember that these fibers control the rate of electrical activity that drives your heart.

In the chest

After the nerve has left the bottom of the neck, it descends into the chest, behind the first and second ribs and in front of the larger blood vessels that extend from the heart. The left vagus nerve runs in front of the arch of the aorta and then sends out its fourth branch, the recurrent nerve. On the opposite side of the body, the right vagus nerve follows a similar path, but passes in front of the right subclavian artery and then sends its fourth branch, the right recurrent nerve. Both recurrent nerves follow a similar path, but on opposite sides of the body. These are the only branches of the nerve that turn and go back up towards the neck.

They transmit motor signals from the brain stem to each of the laryngeal muscles below the vocal cords, which are important for the production of vocal sounds. They are based on tensioning and releasing the vocal cords. We will talk more about how we can use these specific branches to improve the vagus nerve when it is functioning suboptimally. Once the nerves reach the level of the aorta, each of the vagus nerves sends branches to the next pair of organs, the lungs.

The left vagus nerve sends a lung branch to the anterior pulmonary plexus and the right vagus nerve sends a lung branch to the posterior pulmonary plexus. These nerve branches mix with sympathetic neurons, reorganize themselves, then travel to both sides to penetrate the lung. These branches travel to the bronchi and larger branches of the lung to open and close them according to the needs of the body in any situation.

One organ in the thorax that the vagus nerve innervates is often overlooked or forgotten: the thymus. The thymus is an extremely important organ of the immune system. It is located in the mediastinum of the chest, in front of the heart but behind the breastbone. A branch of the vagus makes its way to this nerve to send signals to and from the thymus. The thymus is formed early in our development and is the most important source for the training and growth of our white blood cells.

The reason why this organ is so easily forgotten is that over time it shrinks and is replaced by fatty tissue. This process begins at puberty and can last for many years until early adulthood. I like to think of the thymus as a school for new immune cells, and as the school gets old and deteriorates, the quality of the training through which the white blood cells go decreases.

In the abdominal area

The last section that the vagus nerve penetrates is the organs of the abdomen. These organs are important for digestion, for controlling the immune system and for ensuring that the blood that reaches the rest of our cells does not contain toxins that can negatively affect cell health.

The first abdominal branch of the vagus nerve goes into the stomach. When our body is at rest and digesting, the fibers of the vagus nerve stimulate the abdominal muscles to function. They send signals to the parietal cells to produce and secrete hydrochloric acid (HCI), to the main cells to produce and secrete the digestive enzymes pepsin and gastrin and to the smooth muscle cells of the stomach to move physically and push the food in our stomach into the next section of the digestive tract, the small intestine.

If the vagus nerve is damaged and does not send these important signals to the stomach cells, this leads to problems such as hypochlorhydria or low stomach acidity, which is one of the main causes of many health problems. A sufficiently low pH value (high acidity) is required to activate digestive enzymes and break down food. The optimal pH of the stomach should be around 3.0 in the stomach, with nothing above 5.0 strong enough to activate pepsin and gastrin. A low stomach acid level leads to a less optimal breakdown of food.

A higher pH value in the stomach can also cause unwanted bacteria, viruses, and parasites to find their way into the intestines and wreak havoc in the digestive tract. The second abdominal branch of the vagus goes to the liver. Interestingly, these branches are strongly linked to the feeling of hunger and the desire for certain nutrients. The food we eat first reaches the stomach to be broken down. It then passes into the small intestine, where most of our macronutrients (fats, carbohydrates and amino acids from proteins) are absorbed into the bloodstream.

These nutrients then flow through the portal vein to the liver to filter, process and send signals back to the brain. From the liver, the vagus transmits information to the brain that relates to blood sugar levels, fat intake, and general liver function. The vagus nerve can also transmit information about the amount of bile needed to help digest fats.

The liver has many functions that require vaginal input, including and certainly not limited to the production of bile and salts (the active component of bile), which are then directed to the gallbladder for storage, balancing blood sugar by producing glucose, To control hunger and satiety by measuring fat intake, filtering the blood in the portal vein that brings all the nutrients and toxins from the intestines, and detoxification processes for fat-soluble hormones, neurotransmitters, and toxins from the body in phase 1 and phase 2. The liver is very important for our general well-being and vaginal nutrition is closely linked to maintaining this balance.

The gall bladder is closely connected to the liver. The gallbladder, which is often overlooked by the medical system, is important for the optimal functioning of our body. When the liver produces bile and bile salts, they are sent to the gallbladder for storage to prepare for the next meal. At the next meal, the gallbladder pumps bile into the duodenum (the first part of the small intestine) to transport fats into the bloodstream.

The pump of the gall bladder is mediated by the vagus nerve. From the liver, the vagus branches out to send signals to the gallbladder that activate the smooth muscle cells in its walls to pump bile into the digestive tract. This is in response to a meal that the taste buds (sensory receptors on the tongue) have determined contains fat that should be digested as soon as it reaches the small intestine.

The next branch of the vagus is directed towards the pancreas. Your pancreas is one of the most important glands in your body with an exocrine and an endocrine component. The endocrine pancreas produces and secretes insulin and glucagon directly into the bloodstream to balance the level of glucose in the blood (blood sugar). The exocrine pancreas produces and secretes digestive enzymes through a channel directly into the small intestine.

The three main digestive enzymes of the pancreas are protease, which breaks down proteins into their amino acids, lipase, which breaks down fats from their triglyceride component into free fatty acids and cholesterol, and amylase, which breaks down carbohydrates into simpler sugars.

Vaginal nervation sends signals from the pancreas back to the brain stem and provides information on the status of exocrine and endocrine cells. It also transmits information about food intake from the brain stem to the organ and knows which enzymes are needed for production and release into the bloodstream and digestive tract.

Vaginal innervation is essential for the transmission of this information, as a lack of signaling alters the release of digestive enzymes and reduces the effectiveness of the digestive process. As soon as the vagus nerve moves past the stomach, it forms the celiac plexus, a network formed between the lumbar sympathetic nerves and the parasympathetic fibers of the vagus. This network sends branches to the other organs in the abdomen.

The first organ that is innervated after the celiac plexus is the spleen. The spleen is located on the left side of the body, below the left lung, opposite the liver. Its function is to monitor the bloodstream and activate or deactivate cells of the immune system, depending on what they perceive. At the beginning of our life, both the spleen and the thymus control the immune cell function, but later in life, when the thymus has disappeared, this system is controlled only by the spleen.

The spleen receives messages from the sympathetic branches to activate the inflammatory pathways that intervene in response to physical and biochemical trauma or damage. The parasympathetic branches send signals to stop the inflammatory processes. The vagus nerve modulates a system known as the cholinergic anti-inflammatory pathway, which has a major impact on the spleen.

We will discuss these specific effects in later sections in the context of inflammation. The next branch of the vagus after the celiac plexus moves into the small intestine. Once the food has been broken down by the chemical and physical upheaval in the stomach, it moves to the small intestine. Here it is further processed by pancreatic digestive enzymes and bile to aid digestion. The function of the small intestine is to break down and absorb most of our macronutrients. These include fats, carbohydrates, and proteins (which are ideally broken down into their components, the amino acids).

The bloodstream receives the macronutrients that were absorbed by the lining cells of the small intestine. The morsel that we ingest (which is called chyme at this point in the digestive process) must be pushed along the winding and progression of the small intestine. To do this, the vagus nerve activates the smooth muscle cells of the digestive tract by signaling the extensive network of nerves that line the intestine, the so-called enteric nervous system.

We have an immensely important relationship with the other cells that live in our digestive tracts. I am talking about the symbiotic relationship between our human cells and the bacteria that live in our intestines: The microbiome. The vast majority of our bacterial allies live in our colon, the thicker and shorter part of the digestive tract. Although these bacteria produce many important vitamins, minerals and biochemical basic materials for us, they can also produce many toxins and gases.

We need a system that keeps these bacteria in check and transmits signals to our brain concerning the condition of the digestive tract and microbiome function. So, while the vagus nerve activates smooth muscle cells to push food along the rest of the digestive tract, it is also the main pathway for the microbiome to talk to the brain. The vagus nerve penetrates approximately the first half of the colon, the ascending and transverse part.

The last organ that is penetrated by the vagus nerve is actually two organs, one on each side of the body, the kidneys. These organs have several different functions that are crucial to our health. The kidneys filter the fluid in the form of urine, a combination of uric acid and water, out of the body, which is then passed into the bladder. One of the most important factors influencing this control is blood pressure, which is discussed further in the next chapter.

The vagus nerve is an important controller of kidney function and thus plays an important role in controlling blood pressure. At the end of its course, the vagus nerve does not simply end. Rather, it forms a final plexus with the parasympathctic nerves that originate from the lower end of the spinal cord. These parasympathetic fibers penetrate the second half of the colon, the so-called descending and sigmoid colon, as well as the bladder and the genitals.

The functions of the vagus nerve

A well-functioning UN is crucial to maximizing health and halting the progression of disease. There are many reasons for this and we will go through some of them in this chapter. An optimally functioning body is like a symphony orchestra. In a symphony, each of the different instruments has certain parts to play and optimal harmony can only be achieved when each instrument is focused on its task.

The conductor of the orchestra manages to make sure that no instrument is out of time, as a single mistake can lead to terrible performance. A conductor who does not achieve his goal also leads to a dysfunctional performance. The vagus nerve is the conductor of the symphony orchestra of the human body. It regulates the function of so many different organs and cells in our body, but it can only do so if it is functioning optimally.

He must be able to correctly detect and signal the many organs and cells of the body. Disturbed signaling leads to a lack of harmony in the body and eventually to a state of dysfunction and illness. Let us break down all the different functions that the conductor of the human body orchestra, the vagus nerve, performs.

Sensation of the ear skin

As discussed in the previous chapter, the first branch of the vagus nerve is the auricular branch, which is specifically involved in the perception of the skin of the pinna, the tragus and the external auditory canal of the ear. The function of this branch is purely sensory, allowing us to feel pressure, touch, temperature, and humidity in the central part of each ear. This is clinically relevant and very important as this is one of the most important areas through which the UN can be stimulated using techniques such as acupuncture.

The swallowing of food

When you eat a meal, the last thing you think about is swallowing with every bite and interrupting your breathing reflex so that you do not suffocate. This important task is performed by the vagus nerve. The second branch of the VN (the pharyngeal branch) controls the activation of five muscles of the pharynx: the three constricted muscles at the back of the throat and two other muscles that connect the throat and the soft palate (the soft tissue at the back of the roof of the mouth).

These muscles are involved in the pharyngeal phase of swallowing, in which chewed food is pushed towards the larynx and oesophagus while it is held out of the trachea, leaving the airways free of food. This branch of the UN also manages the active motor component of the gag reflex. Clinically, this is important because poor vagus nerve function leads to coughing and a change in the function of the gag reflex. We can use this reflex to strengthen the VN through active exercises and activation of the gag reflex.

Management of the respiratory tract and vocal cords

With every breath, are you aware of the effort required to keep your upper airways open? The muscles involved in this process are also involved in the production of your voice. If you have ever wondered which nerve is responsible for making verbal communication with your fellow human beings possible, it is the vagus!

The third and fourth branches of the UN are the laryngeus superior and the recurrent nerve. The laryngeus superior is responsible for the muscles above the vocal cords, while the recurrent nerve branch is responsible for the muscles below the vocal cords. The laryngeus superior carries motor information to some muscles of the larynx and controls the vocal pitch.

The suboptimal function of the laryngeus superior leads to a change in pitch. A chronically hoarse voice or a slightly tiring, monotone voice is a sign of a poor vagal tone (signaling ability) in this branch of the nerve. Irritation of this nerve can also lead to severe coughing and aspiration (i.e. food or drink that enters the respiratory tract due to the impaired function of the vocal cords).

The recurrent nerve branch carries motor information to the muscles under the vocal cords, so that sounds can be formed by opening, closing and tensioning the vocal cord structures. It also has a sensory component that carries information from the esophagus, trachea and the inner mucous membranes of these structures. Dysfunction of these nerves leads to hoarseness, loss of voice and breathing difficulties during physical activity.

These laryngeal muscles control the opening, closing, and function of the airways. Any breathing or speech disorder can, therefore, be attributed to reduced function and tension of the vagus nerve. Breathing and the muscle tone of the airways are of utmost importance for vagal function. Any chronic obstruction of a clear and well-functioning airway affects the function and signaling of feedback from these muscles, which negatively affects the function of your vagus nerve.

Respiration control

What about respiration? Well, the vagus also plays a role in controlling this important task. The lung branch of the UN runs to the pulmonary plexus, connects to the sympathetic nervous system and penetrates the trachea and bronchi of both lungs. The vagus component is a sensory nerve that transmits information about lung expansion and oxygen and carbon dioxide levels to the brain.

In the lungs, the activation of the vagus nerve slows down the breathing rate and deepens the breath. During the resting and digestion phase, breathing tends to be deeper and comes from the diaphragm rather than from the extra muscles for breathing, so the respiratory frequency tends to be lower. When a person moves from a fighting or fleeing state to a resting and digestion phase, a slow and deep breathing rate activates the vagus nerve and stimulates the relaxation reflex.

The vagus tension is necessary to open the airways in the throat, larynx, and trachea. The throat and larynx muscles are stimulated by the motor components of the VN. The suboptimal activity of these neurons can lead to airway congestion, as occurs in chronic obstructive pulmonary disease (COPD) and obstructive sleep apnea. Both diseases are a sign of low vagal tension and the need to activate the vagus nerve. I would even go so far as to say that the obstruction of the airways can be a potential cause of the vagus nerve dysfunction.

Heart rate control

Your heart beats to transport nutrient- and oxygen-rich blood to each of your cells and to transport toxins to the organs that can dispose of them. The UN plays an important role in keeping your heart rate in a comfortable range when your body is not under stress. Without the UN, our hearts would not function within the range of its optimal rate.

The vagus nerve is directly connected to the sinus node, which sends electrical signals to the two atria (the thinner chambers at the top of the heart). It is also directly connected to the atrioventricular node, which controls the pumping rate and contraction pressure of the ventricles (the two thicker, lower chambers of the heart). In times of struggle or flight, the sympathetic nervous system activates the heart to increase the pumping rate and contraction pressure in the two ventricles.

When the stress factor is over, the rest and digestion phase takes over and the body moves towards a vagal activation phase. At this point, the parasympathetic fibers of the VN slow down the heart rate and actively reduce the pressure of the pumping contractions. These fibers reduce activity in the heart, allowing the heart to rest and recover from stressful situations and difficult activation.

Maintenance of an optimal blood pressure

Blood pressure is a determining factor for the amount of fluid present in the bloodstream. The kidneys serve to filter fluid and toxins from the body and are therefore the body's most important blood pressure manager. The vagus nerve transmits information to and from the kidneys to control the flow of water and fluids within the renal corpuscles, the kidney's basic filtering unit, and thus controls the body's overall blood pressure. When the body is under stress, signals from the blood vessels (especially the carotid gland) are transmitted back to the kidneys via the brain stem and via the vagus and sympathetic nerves.

The kidneys then constrict their blood vessels and increase blood pressure by reducing the amount of water filtered from the bloodstream. When the body is relaxed, signals from the carotid gland tell the kidneys to filter out more water and dilate the blood vessels to lower blood pressure. Hormones are also closely linked to this process and work in conjunction with the vagus and sympathetic nerves.

However, the immediate control is via the nerves and the slow, gradual control is determined by the hormones. High blood pressure is a very common diagnosis and medication is often prescribed to control these levels. High blood pressure can be a sign of over-activation of stress hormones of the adrenal glands and the stress reaction mediated by the sympathetic nerves. It is also a very common sign of vagus nerve dysfunction and poor vagus tension.

Control of the many liver functions

The vagus nerve transmits much important information to and from the liver and manages its nearly 500 tasks. In this section, I will only discuss some of the most commonly known functions. The liver regulates the blood flow in the body. In times of stress, when the body switches to escape or fight mode, the blood flow is pushed towards the arms and legs to increase muscle activation and allow us to fend off an attack or flee from it. Blood flow in the liver decreases because digestion and blood filtration are not a priority for survival during this stressful event.

When the body is relaxed and in the resting and digestion phase, the activation of the vagus nerves and the blood flow to the liver increase. During this time, digestion, filtration of the blood and other functions are prioritized for cell growth. The vagus nerve also controls the cells in the liver, which are responsible for the production of bile and bile salts and the transport of bile to the gallbladder and small intestine. These cells, called cholangiocytes, are active and increase bile flow into the gallbladder when the vagus nerve is active.

Bile performs several functions for the liver and the body. The liver detoxifies fat-soluble toxins in a two-stage process and produces a water-soluble waste product that must be released. Bile retains these harmless toxins, which are ready to be released from the body via the digestive tract via our stool. The stool is only one of three ways in which waste products are released. The other methods of waste disposal are either as urine through the kidneys or as sweat through the skin.

Bile salts, the effective component of bile, also play a role. When bile is released into the small intestine, it releases waste products and bile salts. Bile salts are needed to transport triglycerides (fat molecules) from the digestive tract, through the enterocytes (the cells lining the small intestine) and into the bloodstream. Without being accompanied by bile salts, fats cannot be absorbed, which is bad because fats and cholesterol have numerous vital functions in the body. This also leads to fatty stools.

The role of the vagus nerve in this function is to activate cholangiocytes and to open the bile flow from the liver to the gall bladder and from the gall bladder to the small intestine, ensuring that fat can be absorbed by enterocytes.

Activation of the emptying of the gall bladder

Once the liver has produced bile and the cholangiocytes have sent it to the gallbladder, it is stored and matures like a good wine until it is needed. When we eat a meal, the taste buds in the tongue and the rest of the mouth send signals to the brain and let our body know about the macronutrients it perceives as part of each bite and the whole of the snack or meal.

When the central nervous system indicates that fats are being consumed, the vagus nerve signals the liver and gallbladder that bile is soon needed. Upon receiving this signal, the gallbladder activates the smooth muscle cells in its lining and pumps the bile through the bile duct into the small intestine to assist in fat digestion. Without this vagus nerve signal, the gallbladder remains full and does not pump out the necessary bile. This is a condition known as obstructive cholestasis.

A common procedure performed in hospitals and clinics is the removal of the gallbladder, the so-called cholecystectomy. The operation to remove a gallbladder due to obstructions, such as gallstones, is often the first option for patients who begin to experience pain associated with obstructive cholestasis.

Unfortunately, most patients do not have the opportunity to determine the cause of this disease. Gallstones are a painful problem that can affect the gall bladder. Gallstones form in the gallbladder after a long period of low vagus nerve function, which would prevent the gallbladder from pumping out enough bile and bile salts.

When bile salts remain in the gallbladder for a long time, they begin to crystallize and form stones. This tends to happen when there is a lack of UN activation and is an early sign of dysfunction in this nerve. Clinical practice has shown that in early cases of this disease gallstones can be excreted when the vagus nerve starts to function at a higher level.

Performing some of the exercises and therapies for vagus nerve activation that we will discuss in later chapters can be very useful for those dealing with gallbladder pain due to cholestasis and gallstone formation.

Control of hunger and satiety

Saturation is reached when our brain receives signals from the vagus nerve. To become saturated, we need signals from the liver to indicate that we have enough fat, protein, and carbohydrates in our body. The metabolism of carbohydrates and fats takes place in the liver. Concerning carbohydrate metabolism, the following control is mediated by the vagus nerve:

When blood sugar levels gradually drop, afferent vagal fibers in the liver increase activity and signal the brain that the liver cells need more carbohydrates. However, this pathway does not signal sudden changes in blood glucose; these are directly perceived in the brain. A hormone called glucagon-like peptide 1 (GLP-1) is released by the small intestine in response to elevated blood sugar levels, which the body translates as saturation. Falling GLP-1 levels signal the vagus nerve, which in turn controls a slow reduction in blood sugar.

Many pharmaceutical companies now produce drugs that work in the GLP-1 pathway to relieve hunger, but this can be controlled in the body by activating the vagus nerve. The vagus nerve offers another route to feelings of satiety. After eating, vagal afferent neurons send information to the brain about the amount of fats that have entered the liver, especially triglycerides and linoleic acid. This activates vagus nerve function and sends a signal to the brain, which creates a feeling of satiety and the desire to stop eating.

An underactive vagus nerve may not be able to send this signal effectively, resulting in persistent feelings of hunger, lack of satiety and excessive eating during the meal. When the UN works effectively, it takes less than 15 to 20 minutes for you to feel full after a meal. If you know someone who lacks the feeling of satiety and whose hunger persists even after a large meal, they probably have UN dysfunction.

Regulation of the blood sugar and insulin levels

Insulin resistance and type II diabetes grow at excessive rates. Obesity and the aptly named "diabesity" - simultaneous diabetes and obesity - are major symptoms of an unhealthy lifestyle. Weight problems and problems with blood sugar levels are important signs that something in your body is working suboptimally. In times of stress, our body shifts its balance towards the sympathetic nervous system and releases more of the adrenal stress hormones, especially cortisol.

The primary effect of cortisol is to increase blood sugar by stimulating a process called gluconeogenesis, in which new glucose is produced from the fats and proteins stored in the liver. In short intervals, the use of the sympathetic nervous system is important to keep us alive and survive.

This combat or escape system was created in response to external threats to our survival. Remember that our ancestors had to run from a saber-toothed tiger. As the stress factor in this situation approaches, our bodies must switch to survival mode. We must either fight the threat or flee and run as fast as possible.

To facilitate fight or flight reactions, our skeletal muscles require substantial energy-producing resources, preferably the fastest and most accessible way to produce cellular energy that would enable us to survive the threat. For short-term fuel, our body can quickly produce glucose by using gluconeogenesis and sending it through the bloodstream.

The sympathetic nervous system quickly shifts the blood flow towards the muscles of the arms and legs to make us overly strong and fast as it shifts it away from the digestive tract and kidneys. We are then able to use our muscles effectively to fight the threat or run away as fast as possible. The problem with this system is that it is often active for longer than is strictly necessary.

Under the chronic stress we experience at work and home with our finances, relationships, friends and family, and due to biochemical stressors, our bodies tend to stay in a fighting or flight state much longer than necessary. We do not return to the resting and digestive state in which the parasympathetic recovery system is mainly active.

The inability to retreat causes the liver to continuously produce glucose, which in the long run leads to higher blood sugar levels. In response to a high blood sugar level, the pancreas is activated to produce insulin. Insulin is the messenger substance that signals each of our cells to take up glucose from the blood and produce energy from it.

Exercises to activate the vagus nerve

In this chapter, I will discuss each of the active exercises and practices that you can do to activate your vagus nerve without buying expensive equipment. Much of the research on this topic shows that regularly performed active exercises are just as effective as (if not more effective than) instruments for stimulating the UN.

The practices and exercises discussed in this chapter all prove to be effective in increasing vagal tone. It is important to remember that the vagus nerve is not just a parasympathetic signaling nerve: the VN has four separate components, each of which can be stimulated to allow optimal signaling and activation of the other three components. These components are:

1. Skin sensation from the central part of the ear

2. Motor innervation of pharynx and larynx
3. Parasympathetic innervation of the heart, lungs and other organs
4. Afferent vagus neurons that send signals back to the brain via visceral fibers.

Consider these four components as we go through these exercise options

Breathing exercises

The first and most effective way to positively influence your vagus nerve is to learn how to breathe properly. Simply put, fast and shallow chest breathing is a sign of stress that activates the sympathetic branch, while slow and deep abdominal breathing is a sign of calm that activates the vagus nerve.

The vast majority of us have not learned to breathe properly. We have subconsciously adjusted ourselves to forget the correct mechanisms of breathing. Correct breathing patterns are directly linked to the functioning of the autonomic nervous system and altered breathing patterns tell the body that it is under stress. This fact is reinforced when one considers that the average person takes about 23,040 breaths per day.

If we want to learn the best, most efficient and effective way to breathe, we need to look to leaders and examples who live among us. Consider some of the greatest vocal and instrumental musicians of our time. If you have ever attended a concert or opera, you have probably noticed that exceptional singers and instrumentalists can sing a whole range of songs without much of a break. Opera singers are some of the most effective breathers on the planet because they have learned to control the function of their diaphragm while holding the vibration of their singing muscles.

You too can learn to create an optimal breathing pattern that can signal to your body that you are not under stress, allowing optimal signaling via the vagus nerve and the parasympathetic nervous system. Several research studies have shown that slow breathing exercises are very effective in improving heart rate variability (HRV). One study showed that slowing the respiratory rate down to six full breaths per minute for five minutes was effective in immediately increasing HRV.

If this is individualized, the effect on HRV is even more effective. Determining the optimal breathing rate that feels right for you individually has the greatest positive effect on your HRV level.

Here are simple steps to perform this exercise:

1. Sit upright without your back leaning against anything.

2. Exhale completely to remove all air from the lungs.

3. Place your right hand on your chest and your left hand on your belly, just above your navel.

4. Breathe deeply through your nose for five to seven seconds and let only your stomach rise (feel only your left hand rising).

5. Hold your breath for two to three seconds.

6. Exhale through your mouth for six to eight seconds and let your stomach sink (feel only your left hand fall).

7. Hold your breath for two to three seconds without air entering your lungs.

8. Repeat steps 4 to 7 as often as you like or for a certain time.

Take five minutes a day to practice deep abdominal breathing yourself and your body will thank you for it. For best results, you should do this exercise several times a day, especially in times of stress. Just one minute of concentrated focus on slow and deep breathing can have a significant positive effect on mood, stress levels, and overall health. Concentrate your attention on inhaling through your nose and not through your mouth to make this exercise even more effective when you do it.

Breathing patterns during sleep

Now that we have talked about the importance of optimal breathing patterns when awake, it is time to ask: What about sleep? The average person requires between seven and eight hours of restful sleep per night, during which time he takes about 7,200 breaths. This is important because almost a third of our breaths are taken while we are not awake. We can train ourselves to breathe optimally when we are conscious and in control of our actions, but what happens when we sleep?

Research has shown that we tend to fall back on bad breathing habits during sleep. This is important, as airway congestion can negatively affect our health and physical function if we are not fully conscious. Obstructive sleep apnea is a growing problem and must be addressed if we are to improve our health. I have personally studied sleep apnea and know that many people have symptoms, although they may not realize it is happening.

It was only when I got married that I was made aware of the subject. My wife pointed out to me that in the middle of the night I would not breathe for no reason and also snored quite a lot. This had a negative effect on my sleep and as you can imagine, it sent a stress signal to my body, as it essentially suffocated several times during the night. It also indicated that my vagus nerve was not functioning optimally.

The symptoms improved as I eliminated much of my excess body fat, but they still appeared from time to time, especially when I was extremely tired before falling asleep. It was a problem until a friend of mine introduced me to a great tool. This tool is called tape and I use it all the time now.

Mouth tape involves sticking a piece of tape over the mouth to close the lips while sleeping. This essentially forces the airflow to go through your nose while you sleep. No single tool has been more effective in improving my breathing patterns, which has allowed me to sleep deeper and more restful and has reduced my allergies.

When we breathe through the mouth, it is much more difficult to use the diaphragm to breathe, but when we breathe through the nose, it is completely normal and habitual. HRV studies have shown that we improve vagus nerve function when we breathe through the nose, as opposed to the pathological form through the mouth. Active breathing exercises during the day and oral tape at night are a powerful combination of tools to improve your breathing patterns both day and night.

First-class sleep

We all know how important it is to have a good night's sleep. Here are some tools that you can use as part of a bedtime routine to increase your chances of a healthy, restful night's sleep. It has been shown that restful sleep improves autonomic balance through heart rate variability studies.

Avoid blue light in the evening

The wavelengths of light change throughout the day and our body has adapted to its signals. When the sun rises in the morning, the light is quite warm in the red/yellow wavelengths. Around noon the light is much bluer and sharper. In the evening, when the sun goes down, the light changes back to a red/yellow tone. These are the signals with which our body tells us the current time of day, as well as the hormones and signals that we should secrete at certain times.

Our screens, including laptop, television, telephone, and tablet, all emit a blue wavelength of light. When we look at our screens every night just before we go to bed, we send our bodies the signal that it is noon. This slows down the release of melatonin, an important hormone that helps us relax and fall asleep deeply. Some devices today have built-in blue light filters, but most do not.

To reduce blue light exposure while you are still using equipment and monitors in the evening, you can do the following:

- Enable Night Shift on your Apple devices.

- Download the Twilight app to Android devices.

- Download f.lux or Iris to your computer (Mac or Windows).

- Use blue-blocking sunglasses when sitting in front of the TV.

Instead of looking at the screen at night, I recommend that you read a physical book or spend device-free time with your loved ones or friends, as social bonding is another great way to improve vagus nerve function.

Switch off the electronics at night

One of the best things I ever did for my health was to cancel my cable TV subscription. It forced me to stop watching TV at night. Since then, I have taken steps to reduce electronic use in the evening and at night and get noticeably better sleep. If you charge your devices such as cell phones or tablets in another room, turn off Wi-Fi routers with automatic timers, and even use your devices in flight mode, you won't be able to use them at night.

Do not eat or drink too late

Nightly toilet breaks often break the restful sleep. When you eat or drink later in the evening, you prepare your body to go to the toilet at night. Instead, you should take your last meal at least two hours before going to bed and your last sip of water at least one hour before going to bed. Your waist and energy level will thank you the next day!

Love your habitat

Sleeping in a clean, organized space is essential to improve your sleep quality and health. If your bedroom is a mess, you can't help but think about the cleaning and organization that needs to be done before going to bed.

This negative energy creeps into your mind and makes your sleep restless, which simply means additional stress for the body and is an easy way to shut down the parasympathetic recovery system at night. Make sure that you keep your room clean and organized regularly, as this has a direct impact on your mood and energy level. I recommend reading Marie Kondo's books on cleaning.

Cold exposure

Have you ever jumped into a lake or swimming pool and then found that the water is icy and freezes you to your core? Your teeth start chattering and your body starts shaking uncontrollably. Your breath is also completely out of control. Your breathing is extremely shallow and you cannot rest your diaphragm sufficiently to calm down and breathe deeply. As you can imagine, this scenario is ideal to activate your sympathetic nervous system and the fight or flight reaction.

Your body struggles to survive in the short term and this has a direct impact on how your body reacts. Your breath becomes shallow and fast, your heart rate increases and your body does not want to digest optimally during this time. All these short-term efforts are for survival.

It may surprise you that this leads to the amazing effect of activating the parasympathetic nervous system in the long term.

Continuous acute exposure to cold or cryotherapy teaches you to regulate your breathing, which has an overall positive effect on vagus activation and significant anti-inflammatory effects throughout the body.

Regular exposure to cold is one of the best and easiest ways to activate and heal a failed vagus nerve. The easiest way to integrate this into your life is to take a cold shower. A great tip that I give to many people around me is to shower normally and at the end of the shower to set the temperature as cold as possible and let the water splash on your head and neck at the last minute. It will initially be shocking for the body and will change the way you breathe.

During this time your goal is to work on controlling your breath and doing as many deep abdominal breaths as possible. If you can train your body to breathe in the cold, your vagus nerve will become very strong and your body will have an optimally functioning parasympathetic nervous system and vagus nerve. If this minute becomes easier, you can add a minute or two of cold exposure per week until your entire shower is spent in freezing water and a huge smile appears on your face!

Humming or singing

Another way to activate the vagus nerve is to stimulate and use the voluntary muscles it signals. By activating these muscles, you stimulate the brainstem centers that send signals through the vagus, not only the muscle control centers but also all the others around it. By humming and singing, you can activate the muscles of the larynx, which receives signals directly from the laryngeus superior and the VN recurrent nerve.

They allow our vocal cords to tighten and loosen up due to muscle tension, which gives us a pitch in our voices. When we practice buzzing deep in the throat, we activate and vibrate these muscles and stimulate the vagus to send these signals. Perhaps you are aware of the sacred Hindu syllable "Om" which is used to create a deep vibration in the throat when it is played out loud.

The vibration of "Om", which is said to vibrate on the resonance plane of God, has a strong spiritual affiliation in the practice of Hinduism. Other cultures use simple words like amine, ant, and amen, but they all seem to mean the Word of God.

When you sing the word and use this frequency, the laryngeal muscles of the neck and vocal cords are stimulated, which allows the stimulation of the motor fibers of the VN. If done long enough and with enough force, it can be an effective way to stimulate the other signaling components of the nerve. It allows us to control our breath, slow down our thoughts, and concentrate on extremely deep relaxation.

It has been shown to improve digestion and inflammation in the body. Buzzing or singing the word "Om" before a meal can be a good way to calm down, adapt to the universe and stimulate the activity of the vagus nerves in the digestive tract and other visceral organs. If you practice "Om" during other times, including after a stressful event, it is a valuable tool to lower stress levels and increase sympathetic activation after that stressful event.

There are other words for humming or singing that can actively stimulate these muscles and improve vagus nerve signaling, but "Om" is one that I have personally found to be very effective because the vibration of the neck muscles during exercise is very obvious.

Activating the gag reflex

Following the humming and singing, the activation of the gag reflex is another way to stimulate the muscles stimulated by the UN. Also known as the throat reflex, this reflex, which involves a cycle of nerve activation to function optimally, is necessary to protect us from suffocation. When an object we do not know enters our mouth and touches our soft palate (the soft part on the back of the roof of the mouth), a very rapid sensory signal is sent through the ninth cranial nerve to the brainstem and the motor aspect of three different cranial nerves.

The first of these nerves is the pharyngeal branch of the vagus, which immediately contracts the three pharyngeal muscles at the back of the throat to prevent the object from penetrating further into the body and possibly getting stuck in the airways. The fifth cranial nerve and the twelfth cranial nerve are also stimulated and cause the jaw to open and push the tongue forward to push the object out. Voluntary activation of the gag reflex sends an immediate signal to the vagus and the other nerves so that they can signal quickly and optimally.

The best time for this is twice a day while brushing your teeth. With the toothbrush, you can touch the soft palate and stimulate this reflex. This is a great and simple option that is known to have a direct effect on UN signaling. Since we have a series of cranial nerves on both sides of our body, it is necessary to stimulate the soft palate on both sides to get the full benefit of this exercise.

Gurgles

When I was a child, my father often encouraged me to gargle with saltwater in the morning and evening after brushing my teeth, as he did every day all his life. He always told me that it was good for my health. I still didn't take it seriously and didn't think about it any further. Interestingly enough, he had an idea about something. I should have known because he is a very healthy seventy-year-old. Gargling is the process of taking a sip of water into the back of your throat and throwing it around with force.

It requires the activation of the three pharyngeal muscles at the back of the throat and is, therefore, another method of stimulating the vagus nerve by muscle activation. As my father always reminded me, twice a day after brushing my teeth is a good way to use this tool easily. For best results, it is best to gargle with extra force until your eyes start watering. When your vagus "ignites", it actively sends signals from its brainstem nuclei, which activate some neighboring nuclei as they become stronger.

In this case, the upper salivary nucleus is stimulated, which causes the glands around the eyes to produce fluid that turns into tears. If you gargle hard enough to make you cry, you'll do it right and have a great effect on your vagus nerve. It is also a good option to add a little salt to the water, such as pink Himalayan salt.

The gargling of saltwater has been shown to have an antibacterial effect and can help remove some unwanted bacteria from the mouth and upper airways. Using essential oils, such as oregano oil in water, is another great option with very similar effects.

Mindfulness Practice

Before starting a task, do you take a moment to sit still, close your eyes and focus your attention? Make sure that you are 100% committed to the task at hand?

When you are resting, do you take a moment to be grateful for your surroundings? Mindfulness is just that: taking the time and making an effort to pay attention to what you are doing and what is happening around you.

Many of us jump from task to task or extinguish one fire after another without paying attention to what is going on around us. We are so caught up in our minds that the attention is focused on a single task and full attention is drawn to it; it feels like a waste of time and effort.

Consciousness exercise means to perform each task with 100 percent of your attention focused on that task to achieve your maximum performance. It means taking in your environment, being aware of everything that brought you to this very moment and being grateful for it. The ability to practice mindfulness cannot occur when we are stressed or angry and in pain. Our sympathetic nervous system tends to diminish our attention and prevent us from focusing on what we are doing.

When you actively practice mindfulness throughout the day, you focus on your breath and how to achieve each task. This shifts the balance towards the parasympathetic nervous system and allows the UN to do its work. Attention to a task means doing one thing with full attention and finishing it before moving on to the next task. Conscious eating allows you to feel full and not overeat. Mindful relaxation allows you to feel rested and rejuvenated faster than you can imagine.

All of this requires the vagus nerve to be active and engaged, as we need to be able to rely on it for our body to rest, digest and recover. Multitasking is exactly the opposite of mindfulness. Being attentive to what I do, what I eat and feel as each task approaches was the most positive change I have made in my life.

It is by far the main reason why my health prognoses have become more and more positive. It has been a great pioneer for me and countless others around me and I am sure that it can also bring about profound positive changes in your life.

Meditation

Meditation is similar to the application of mindfulness. It is the art of watching your breath and teaching your attention not to follow every thought that comes into your mind. Our brain is designed to recognize and form dynamic, ingenious connections between our thoughts and actions. Meditation teaches us to listen to our hearts and focus on our breath by learning to become observers of our thoughts and not victims of their fluidity. Instead of discussing the countless methods of meditation, I would like to talk about their benefits.

Studies on heart rate variability have shown that meditation has a significant positive effect on the function of the vagus nerve because while we meditate, our attention is focused on our breath. There are many different types of meditation, but those that focus on the breath are usually the best for improving HRV levels. These include breath meditation, loving kindness, Vipassana and mindfulness meditation.

For beginners, I recommend using audio meditations with instructions on YouTube or via an app on your mobile phone.

Laughter and social connectedness

If you knew that more laughter would improve your health, would you do it more often? Remember the last time you had a good laugh with friends. Did you feel good for the next few hours? Did you sleep better that night? Did you wake up the next morning feeling good?

Continuous research shows time and again that laughter and laughter yoga are very effective in improving mood and heart rate variability. We tend to use our membranes when we laugh with strength and joy, and in turn, we exercise control over our breathing rate and ensure that we can normalize our breathing patterns. This is a training session for the vagus nerve.

To improve the function of the vagus nerve, it is a great and very pleasant way to make powerful laughter a regular event. I make a point of watching funny videos or going to comedy shows as often as possible to feel socially connected and enjoy the health benefits of laughter. Laughter yoga classes in your area, regular meetings with friends to share funny stories and a comedy movie are good ways to laugh more.

Social connectedness is directly related to this, as we tend to laugh out loud when we are around others, especially friends and family. Social connectedness is one of the biggest factors influencing health and can be as important as the food you eat.

People want to be with other people. When we feel lonely and separated from others, both our mood and our health are negatively affected. We tend to enjoy the company of others and prefer face-to-face conversations with real people. When we are with others, we tend to laugh more, smile more and feel more relaxed.

We feel even better when we spend time with people with whom we agree and share values. Recently I was able to take my family to a city festival, which was an amazing experience. The beautiful nature and surroundings were combined with spending time with local people who shared the same values as I did.

If you are feeling lonely, depressed or just disconnected, find a way to spend time with others and connect with people who have similar values to yourself. If physical fitness is an important value, you should join a gym or join a yoga class with friends. If communication is an important value for you, join a Toastmasters group and practice your public speaking skills with supportive and like-minded people. If you value having a good time with others, go to a movie or dinner with friends so you can talk and have a great time.

There are 7 billion people on the planet and countless activities and interactions that allow you to connect with these people. It is believed that we laugh less as we get older, but the healthiest people I know care about laughing more.

And in the blue zones, the regions around the world with the highest longevity rates (many people live over 100 years but are still physically active), social connectedness is a common theme. So get out there, enjoy social experiences with those around you, meet new people, exchange funny stories and laugh as loudly and as often as you can. That's an order!

Daily exercise or sport

Our bodies are made to move. Muscles are some of the most important and overlooked organs in the body, and muscle cells help us best to balance our blood sugar and body fat levels - when we use them. The problem is that most of us sit for a very long time every day and do not move. Then we sit in the car and sit on the couch and repeat this lack of exercise every day.

Exercising a certain amount of physical activity, preferably one that increases the heart rate by increasing physical stress for a short period, helps to improve parasympathetic nerve activity. There are times when both the sympathetic and parasympathetic systems can be activated and recovery after exercise is one of these.

During recovery, we optimize our breathing pattern, which increases the signal to the muscles of the airways to increase patency and cause the heart to get stronger and release more blood with each pump. It also allows us to regularly return to a parasympathetic state.

If you move your muscles and get your body to do things that put a strain on it every day, the body will learn how to recover from the stress faster while helping you balance energy levels and macronutrient fuel sources. Use your muscles to get your body to do things, preferably outdoors.

Solar radiation

Sunlight during the day is directly related to sleep. Our body is genetically programmed to work based on the amount and type of sunlight that enters our eyes and skin. It has a direct influence on how we function on a cellular level. When we spend an entire day under artificial lighting with limited sunlight, we deprive our cells of optimal signaling and function.

Exposure to light during the day is directly related to improved HRV levels. Our eyes and skin prefer to receive signals of red, infrared and yellow wavelengths during sunrise and sunset, while they prefer blue, green, violet and ultraviolet light during the middle of the day. Solar radiation does this naturally, while our workplaces, cars, and homes do not, at least not yet. Circadian lighting technology is being developed by many companies at the time of this book.

Since sunlight is directly related to HRV levels, it is highly recommended that you go outside every day and get direct sunlight on your skin. It is even better if you do this at several different times of the day. The best times to go outside are within 30 minutes of sunrise (two to three times a day) and within 30 minutes of sunset. It is even better to spend the whole day outside whenever possible. You are far less likely to burn your skin during the day if your body feels the sunrise and is prepared for the UV light we experience during the day.

BONUS: 5 effective exercises to activate your vagus nerve

Bonus #1: Use of breathing to relieve pain

You can learn to use breathing exercises to shift your focus away from pain. The human mind processes one thing at a time. If you concentrate on the rhythm of your breathing, you are not concentrating on the pain. The moment we expect pain, most of us tend to stop breathing and hold our breath. Holding the breath activates the fight, flight and freeze reaction, it tends to increase the feeling of pain, stiffness, fear or anxiety. You can proceed as follows: Inhale deeply through your stomach (i.e. expand your diaphragm), count to five, pause and then exhale slowly through a small hole in your mouth. At rest, most people take about 10 to 14 breaths per minute.

To enter the parasympathetic/relax-ing/healing mode, it is ideal to reduce the breath to 5 to 7 times per minute. Exhaling through the mouth instead of the nose makes breathing more conscious and helps you to control your breath more easily. As you reduce your breaths per minute and switch to the parasympathetic mode, your muscles will relax and your worries and fears will fall away. The oxygen supply to your body cells increases and helps to pro-duce endorphins, the body's feel-good hor-mones.

Tibetan monks have practiced "conscious breathing" for decades, but there is nothing mysterious about it. You can improve your experience by imagining that you inhale love and exhale gratitude. These ancient techniques also improve memory, combat depression, lower blood pressure or heart rate, and strengthen the immune system, all for free!

Bonus #2: Singing "Om"

An interesting study was conducted by the International Journal of Yoga in 2011, comparing OM chanting with the pronunciation of "sss" and a state of rest to determine whether singing is more stimulating to the vagus nerve. The study found that singing was more effective than either the "sss" or the resting state. Effective "OM" singing is associated with the experience of a vibrational sensation in the area of the ears and the whole body. It is expected that such a feeling is also transmitted through the auricular branch of the vagus nerve and causes a limbic (HPA axis) deactivation.

How you can sing

Hold the vowel ("o") part of the "OM" for 5 seconds and then move to the consonant ("m") part for the next 10 seconds. Continue singing for 10 minutes. Take a deep breath and finish with gratitude.

Bonus#3: Cold water

Physical exercise leads to an increase in sympathetic activity (HPA axis - fight/escape and stress response), together with parasympathetic withdrawal (rest, digestion, healing, immune system), resulting in higher heart rates. Studies have shown that immersing the face in cold water seems to be a simple and efficient means of immediately accelerating parasympathetic reactivation after exercise via the vagus nerve, stimulating the reduction of heart rate, intestinal mobility, and activation of the immune system.

It also works in a non-sporting environment to activate the vagus nerve. The subjects remained seated while immersed in the cold water and bent their heads forward in a pool of cold water. The face was immersed so that forehead, eyes and at least two-thirds of both cheeks were underwater. The water temperature was 10-12 °C.

Bonus #4: Increased saliva flow

The calmer the mind and the deeper the relaxation, the easier it is to stimulate the saliva. If the mouth can produce abundant saliva, you know that the vagus nerve has been stimulated and your body is in parasympathetic mode. To stimulate saliva flow, try to relax and sit on a chair and imagine a juicy lemon.

If your mouth fills with saliva, just rest your tongue in this "bath" (if that doesn't happen, just fill your mouth with a small amount of warm water and leave your tongue in this bath. Just performing the relaxation stimulates the saliva production). Now relax further and feel your hands, feet, hips, neck, and head relax. Breathe deeply into this feeling and stay with it as long as you can.

Bonus #5: Massages

You can stimulate your vagus nerve by massaging your feet and neck along the carotid artery located on either side of the neck. A neck massage can help reduce seizures. A foot massage can help reduce heart rate and blood pressure. A pressure massage can also activate the vagus nerve. These massages are used to help babies gain weight by stimulating intestinal function, which is largely mediated by activation of the vagus nerve.

Closing words

I'm grateful that you took the time to read my work. I hope it inspired you and made you take control of your health again. Now that you understand the nature of the parasympathetic nervous system and the extent to which the vagus nerve transmits information, the power is in your hands to improve its function and regain your health. For some of you, these strategies and protocols will have profound effects that will dramatically improve energy, digestion, inflammation, and pain, while for others it may simply be the first step in the journey. Wherever you find yourself on your health journey, take a moment to commit to being responsible for this knowledge. Share it with those around you - family, friends and perhaps even work colleagues - who need to hear that there are answers to what may be troubling them. I am truly grateful for each reader and I wish you all the best on your journey.

Disclaimer

The implementation of all information, instructions, and strategies contained in this e-book is at your own risk. The author cannot assume any liability for any damages of any kind for any legal reason. Liability claims against the author for material or non-material damages caused by the use or non-use of the information or by the use of incorrect and/or incomplete information are excluded in principle. Any legal and compensation claims are therefore also excluded. This work has been compiled and written down with the utmost care and to the best of our knowledge. However, the author accepts no responsibility for the topicality, completeness, and quality of the information. Printing errors and incorrect information cannot be completely excluded. No legal responsibility or liability of any kind can be assumed for incorrect information provided by the author.

Copyright

Imprint

www.ingramcontent.com/pod-product-compliance
Lightning Source LLC
Chambersburg PA
CBHW050650250726
48662CB00002B/596